الشفاء المحمدي

The Muhammadan Cure

The Modern Science of Prophetic Medicine

A commentary of Ṭib al-Nabī by Abu'l ʿAbbās Jaʿfar b. Muḥammad al-Mustaghfirī (d. 432 AH)

Bilal Muhammad

To my lovely, loving, and beloved parents

Table of Contents

Introduction

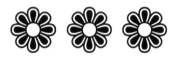

Praise be to Allah, the Healer (*al-Shāfī*), the Protector (*al-Mu'min*), the Provider (*al-Razzāq*), the Extender (*al-Bāṣiṭ*), the Responsive (*al-Mujīb*), the Lover (*al-Wadūd*), and the Giver of Life (*al-Muḥyī*). May His peace and blessings be upon His beloved servant Muḥammad b. ʿAbdullāh, as well as his family and those who followed him.

Allah is our Creator, and He is the Creator of wellness and illness. In times of health, Allah allows us to be delighted by the goodly things that He has provided us. He strengthens us for acts of obedience, which lead to the furtherance of His bounties. In times of illness, Allah tries us and purifies us from the evil deeds that weigh us down. He reminds us of our limitations and our need for Him. In both wellness and illness, Allah deserves our gratitude.

Islam has never advocated for a sole dependence on "pray-it-away" solutions to our worldly ills. Our faith is built on knowledge and intuition, and action is the outward quality of faith. Thus, the Prophet Muḥammad ﷺ, who is the Seal of Prophets, offers us a workable system by which we can organize our lives and our societies. This book will be highlighting some of the dietary and medicinal recommendations made in the Islamic tradition. Some of these recommendations are ethical in nature, while others promote health and wellbeing. It is not enough to simply enjoy our food – rather, we must look at our food with a critical eye. Whatever we put into our body could either be medicine or poison; and a dose of medicine that is too high can produce adverse effects. Likewise, we are also accountable for our actions. We must make sure that our food is *ḥalāl, ṭayyib,* ethically grown, ethically purchased, and eaten with proper table etiquettes. Islam is a process that encompasses all aspects of our lives.

Heart disease, cancer, diabetes, and mental illnesses are all among the leading causes of preventable death today.[1] In many cases, chronic illnesses can be caused by what we eat. Furthermore, a wholesome dietary regimen is a primary form of treatment for such conditions. Strengthening our bodies with the intention of obeying Allah is a form of worship.

Ṭib al-Nabī ("Medicine of the Prophet") is a vast genre of literature. This book reviews only a small sample of this genre, but the results are eye-opening. Much of the

---

[1] "CDC National Health Report Highlights", Center for Disease Control, https://www.cdc.gov/healthreport/publications/compendium.pdf

ancient prescriptions given are consistent with the conclusions of controlled studies being published in medical journals today. *The Muhammadan Cure* contains over 130 references to published studies and articles. This should be no surprise to any Muslim, as the Prophet ﷺ received his message from God Almighty.

My hope is that this work will inspire readers to do further research into this topic. Food-related illnesses and conditions are rampant in the worldwide Muslim community, and our Prophet ﷺ found it important enough to speak on this topic in great detail. A healthy regimen, after all, is a daily commitment, like prayer.

WORDS OF CAUTION

This work is not meant to replace your doctor or your dietician. I encourage you to seek the advice of medical professionals before administering any substances with the intention of treating your illnesses.

Please be aware of any allergies or food intolerances (including lactose intolerance) that you may have. Many *aḥadīth* in this book do not apply to exceptional circumstances.

Medical studies are subject to human error, correlation-causation fallacies; and there are valid differences of opinion in the medical and dietary fields. Thus, readers should be aware that not all research should be taken as fact.

While this book contains many of the "scientific miracles" of our tradition, be advised that the veracity of our Prophet ﷺ is not to be validated solely through scientific observation. These observations are subject to change and error, while the truth of Islam is not. This work should instead be seen as a commentary on and an elucidation of the possible meaning of these reports. Some *aḥadīth* are also not naturalistic in nature, but rather they enter the genre of morality.

ABOUT THE ORIGINAL WORK

The Muhammadan Cure revivifies *Ṭib al-Nabī by Abu'l ʿAbbās Jaʿfar b. Muḥammad al-Mustaghfirī* (d. 1041 CE). Al-Mustaghfirī was a notable Ḥanafī Ashʿarī *ḥadīth* scholar born in Nasaf, Uzbekistan in the fifth Islamic century. The book came to acclaim and prominence among both Sunnī and Shīʿī medieval scholars. It was included in ʿAllāmah al-Majlisī's magnum opus *Biḥār al-Anwār* in the seventeenth century. There are two surviving versions of the book; I used the one preserved in *Biḥār*.

Although the book contains many well-established narrations from the Prophet Muḥammad ﷺ, not all its reports can be classified as *ṣaḥīḥ*. However, according to most scholars, strict *isnād* analyses are necessary only for theology (*ʿaqāʾid*) and law (*aḥkām*). These metrics are often not used in *tafsīr, tārīkh, mawāʿith*, and other supererogatory areas of religion, including *Ṭib*. Secondly, the scientific merit of these *aḥadīth* can be a modern metric for their veracity.

METHODS

I first reviewed the original Arabic of the full *Ṭib al-Nabī* and an existing translation. The book consists of one hundred and fifty-six reports. I selected fifty-eight of the reports that made prescriptive, medicinal statements. Reports that were not included were mostly less relevant to our study.

After selecting the reports, I re-translated them from Arabic to English. I then compared the statements made in these *aḥadīth* to studies published in the U.S National Library of Medicine, the British Journal of Nutrition, the Journal of Epidemiology, the Journal of Dermatology & Dermatologic Surgery, the Journal of Endocrinology & Metabolism, the Journal of Antimicrobial Chemotherapy, the Journal of Nutritional Biochemistry, the Asian Pacific Journal of Cancer Prevention, the Clinical Journal of American Society of Nephrology, the Journal of Food Protection, JAMA Internal Medicine, the Journal of Medical Science and Clinical Research, the Journal of Midwifery and Reproductive Health, and other scientific and dietary journals and articles.

I summarized my findings below each *ḥadīth*. If the current medical findings did not support a *ḥadīth*; or if there were differences of opinion among medical professionals, I mentioned that in the commentary, to avoid confirmation bias.

I also looked up existing Islamic commentaries of some of these reports. I included other relevant *aḥadīth* from established sources in my comments. Any *aḥadīth* that are not from al-Mustaghfirī's work were not bolded. I included ethical, symbolic, and spiritual dimensions to my commentaries, as not all *aḥadīth* are to be looked at exclusively from a naturalist lens.

The book was then reviewed by two licensed medical doctors. I made revisions based on their expert advice.

The *aḥadīth* were then organized into custom chapters.

ABOUT THE AUTHOR

Bilal Muhammad is a teacher and educator based in Toronto, Canada. He is a Senior Fellow at the Berkeley Institute for Islamic Studies, the Regional Manager of Active Aql Inc in Toronto, and a member of the Muslim Debate Initiative. He holds a B.Ed. from the Ontario Institute for Studies in Education at the University of Toronto. He also holds an Honours B.A. in Political Science, History, and the History of Religions from the University of Toronto. He is a former research assistant to Dr. Shafique Virani at the University of Toronto Department of Historical Studies. He has taken courses in Matn Abi Shuja with Shaykh Jamir Meah.

Bilal Muhammad is neither a medical professional nor a licensed dietician. However, he has taught several accredited ministry-inspected courses, including Nutrition and Health (HFA4U) and Food and Culture (HFC3M).

General

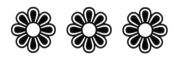

قال رسول الله صلى الله عليه وآله وسلم : ما خلق الله تعالى داء إلا

وخلق له دواء إلا السام .

وقال صلى الله عليه وآله وسلم: الذي انزل الداء انزل الشفاء .

The Messenger of Allah ﷺ said, "Allah the Exalted has not created an illness except that He has created a cure for it, except for death.

He who has sent down the malady has sent down the remedy."

Wellness ontologically precedes illness, as the natural state of the human being is of balance. The origin of every disease is either too much of something, or not enough of something. Thus, a balanced diet is key to avoiding acute and chronic illnesses. One who is ill should actively seek a remedy for his illness via a regimen or a physician.

Allah is the Healer (*al-Shāfī*), and healing is a sign of Him. He is the source of all cures, and a patient only gets better with His permission. Maladies and death are an aspect of this world that represent trial, atonement, and chastisement. An illness may relinquish the sins of a believer whilst being a lesson in patience and humility. Since Islam is not a faith-only creed, it is not enough to pray an illness away. Prayer must be coupled with action.

Allah says in His Book, "Every person shall taste death." (3:85) Whether death is brought about by internal or external factors, death is an unavoidable part of life. Those who trust Allah and perform righteous deeds will enjoy eternal life, while those who do not will be in a wretched state in which there is neither living nor dying (87:13). In this sense, death can be a blessing, because it marks the end of the pain of this world.

The Prophet said, "How astonishing is the affair of the believer! Surely, his whole affair is good for him, and this is not the case for anyone except the believer. If he is prosperous, he is thankful, and that is good for him; and if he is afflicted with adversity, he is patient, and that is good for him." (عجبا لأمر المؤمن إن أمره كله له خير، وليس ذلك

لأحد إلا للمؤمن : إن أصابته سراء شكر فكان خيراً له، وإن أصابته ضراء

صبر فكان خيراً له)

وقال صلى الله عليه وآله وسلم: كل وانت تشتهي وامسك وانت تشتهي.

The Prophet ﷺ said, "Eat when you are craving, and stop while you are [still] craving."

One should stop eating while they are still hungry. It takes approximately twenty minutes for stretch receptors in the stomach to signal the brain that it is full.[2] Thus, one may be full whilst he is still craving. It is therefore important for people to eat slowly, as it will lessen one's overall calorie intake. Obesity is one of the leading causes of preventable death worldwide, and so decreasing portion sizes and increasing physical activity are necessary to a healthy lifestyle.

The narration can also be addressing food waste and gluttony. In poverty and dire situations, it is important to control food intake so that precious resources are not wasted, and that food is properly shared with others.

The Prophet said, "Food for one suffices for two, and food for two suffices for four." (طَعَامُ الْوَاحِدِ يَكْفِي الِاثْنَيْنِ)

(وَطَعَامُ الِاثْنَيْنِ يَكْفِي الْأَرْبَعَةَ)

---

[2] Ann MacDonald, "Why eating slowly may help you feel full faster", Harvard Health Publishing: Harvard Medical School, https://www.health.harvard.edu/blog/why-eating-slowly-may-help-you-feel-full-faster-20101019605

وقال صلى الله عليه وآله وسلم: من قل اكله قل حسابه .

The Prophet ﷺ said, "One who lessens his eating shall have his reckoning lessened."

The overt meaning of this tradition is that the more one eats, the more he will be accountable for on the Day of Resurrection. Indeed, people will be questioned on the ethics of their eating habits, and it is thus vital that a believer only eats that which is *ḥalāl*. Food is furthermore not to be obtained immorally, eaten wastefully, or harmed prior to slaughter.

Since some sins will be accounted for in this life, it is fathomable that some overeating will karmically result in food-related illnesses. A 2016 study published by JAMA Internal Medicine found that restricting calorie intake had a positive affect on the mood, quality of life, sleep, and sexual function of a sample of healthy adults.[3] The sample reported improved mood and general health, healthy weight loss, and better sexual functioning.

The Prophet said, "Fast, and you will become healthier." (صُومُوا تَصِحُّوا) There are many reports on the positive effects of intermittent fasting, but the real benefits of Islamic fasting will be known in the next world.

---

[3] Corby K. Martin et al, "Effect of Calorie Restriction on Mood, Quality of Life, Sleep, and Sexual Function in Healthy Nonobese Adults", JAMA Internal Medicine, https://jamanetwork.com/journals/jamainternalmedicine/fullarticle/2517920

وقال صلى الله عليه وآله وسلم: برد الطعام فان الحار لا بركة فيه .

The Prophet ﷺ said, "Cool the food, for surely, there is no blessing in heat."

This narration advises one to eat food cool rather than scorching hot. One can burn their lips, tongue, gums, or esophagus when eating hot food.

Cooking food at warm temperatures is critical for food safety. Vegetables, however, can lose significant amounts of vitamin C in the cooking process.[4] Eating very hot food could also be harmful to one's mouth or esophagus. One study suggests that frying foods at high temperatures creates harmful compounds. The temperature causes the food to release neo-formed contaminants, including trans fats, which are known to increase the risk of heart disease.[5]

---

[4] Megan Smith, "Are There Nutritional Differences in Hot and Cold Food?", LiveStrong. https://www.livestrong.com/article/546651-nutritional-differences-in-hot-cold-food/
[5] Raj Bhopal et al, "The high-heat food preparation hypothesis", US National Library of Medicine. https://www.ncbi.nlm.nih.gov/pubmed/27776951

وقال صلى الله عليه وآله وسلم : ثلاث لقمات بالملح قبل الطعام

تصرف عن ابن آدم اثنين وسبعين نوعا من البلاء منه الجنون والجذام

والبرص .

The Prophet ﷺ said, "Three morsels of salt before a meal dissuades seventy-two types of calamity from a son of Adam, amongst them are insanity, leprosy, and vitiligo."

A dose of medicine that is too high can be poisonous. This narration recommends three morsels of salt, which is a much smaller quantity than most people consume daily. However, salt certainly has a role in dieting. Salt stimulates taste buds and increases the secretion of saliva. Saliva makes a food more suitable for digestion. Salt also stimulates the motor nerve of the gland, leading to the secretion of digestive juices in the stomach and intestines. Salt helps the intestines absorb water.

A diet that is deficient of salt can stunt muscle growth and bone growth. Hyponatremia occurs when the concentration of sodium in your blood is abnormally low. Sodium is an electrolyte that helps regulate the water that is in and around your cells.

The symptoms of hyponatremia include headache, confusion, and seizures.[6] Furthermore, a 2018 study

---

[6] "Hyponatremia", Mayo Clinic, https://www.mayoclinic.org/diseases-conditions/hyponatremia/symptoms-causes/syc-20373711

found that leprosy patients are more likely to have an electrolyte imbalance.[7]

A diet that is too high in salt can be bad for cardiovascular health. Those with high blood pressure should limit their salt intake.

وقال صلى الله عليه وآله وسلم : لا وجع إلا وجع العين ، ولاهم إلا هم الدين .

The Prophet ﷺ said, "There is no pain but (i.e. like, as severe as) the pain of the eye, and there is no anxiety but the anxiety of debt."

In a 2008 study, results showed that over-indebted individuals with probable clinical depression and/or anxiety showed greater levels of financial strain, used adaptive coping strategies to a lesser extent, and maladaptive coping strategies to a greater extent. Additionally, financial strain, use of maladaptive and emotion-focused coping, age and employment status were significant predictors of mental illness.[8]

---

[7] Prabhakar Singh Bais et al, "A study on the Electrolytes Imbalance in Leprosy Patients in a Tertiary Care Centre", Journal of Medical Science and Clinical Research, http://jmscr.igmpublication.org/home/index.php/current-issue/5298-a-study-on-the-electrolytes-imbalance-in-leprosy-patients-in-a-tertiary-care-center

[8] Holmgren R et al, "Coping and financial strain as predictors of mental illness in over-indebted individuals in Sweden", US National Library of Medicine, https://www.ncbi.nlm.nih.gov/pubmed/30585328

Eating Utensils

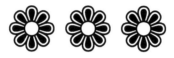

وقال صلى الله عليه وآله وسلم: من استعمل الخشبتين امن من عذاب الكليتين .

The Prophet ﷺ said, "One who uses the two pieces of wood (i.e. the *miswak* and the *khilal* – toothpick) is safe from the affliction of the kidneys."

Poor oral health is common in patients with chronic kidney disease and may contribute to increased deterioration and mortality due to inflammation, infections, protein-energy wasting, and atherosclerotic complications. Uremic patients have higher rates of missing, decayed, and filled teeth than the general population.[9]

Miswak has a plethora of pharmacological properties, including antimicrobial, antioxidant, enzyme inhibitory activity, antiulcer, anticonvulsant, sedative, analgesic, anti-inflammatory, hypoglycemic, hypolipidemic, antiosteoporosis, and antitumor activities.[10]

One controlled study indicates that a miswak-based mouthwash is more affective at removing plaque than other herbal and synthetic mouthwashes.[11] Another study found that miswak-based toothpaste reduced significantly more plaque than toothpaste made from tea tree oil.[12]

The Prophet said, "Had I not found it difficult for my nation, I would have ordered them to use the miswak

[9] Harun Akar et al, "Systemic Consequences of Poor Oral Health in Chronic Kidney Disease patients", Clinical Journal of American Society of Nephrology.
https://cjasn.asnjournals.org/content/6/1/218.full?fbclid=IwAR2etC0T zlrD4m_XlGSjpAhnYeErP0KPO5e4bqT99WVzpRrdOWKOrW9RiJl
[10] Aumeeruddy MZ et al, "A review of the traditional and modern uses of Salvadora persica L. (Miswak): Toothbrush tree of Prophet Muhammad.", US National Library of Medicine.
https://www.ncbi.nlm.nih.gov/pubmed/29196134
[11] Niaz FH et al, "Anti-plaque Efficacy of Herbal Mouthwashes Compared to Synthetic Mouthwashes in Patients Undergoing Orthodontic treatment: A Randomised Controlled Trial." US National Library of Medicine,
https://www.ncbi.nlm.nih.gov/pubmed/30151504
[12] Varma SR et al, "The Antiplaque Efficacy of Two Herbal-Based Toothpastes: A Clinical Intervention." US National Library of Medicine,
https://www.ncbi.nlm.nih.gov/pubmed/29629325

لَوْلاَ أَنْ أَشُقَّ عَلَى أُمَّتِي ـ أَوْ عَلَى النَّاسِ ـ) ''.with every prayer

(لأَمَرْتُهُمْ بِالسِّوَاكِ مَعَ كُلِّ صَلاَةٍ

وقال صلى الله عليه وآله وسلم: تخللوا على اثر الطعام وتمضمضوا

فأنهما مصحة الناب والنواجد .

The Prophet ﷺ said, "Use a toothpick after food, and rinse your mouth, for surely it promotes health in the canine [teeth] and the molars."

While toothpicks can potentially be harmful, the focus of this *ḥadīth* is the removal of food from one's backmost teeth. Molar teeth are often difficult to reach with floss, and wisdom teeth often grow in incorrectly, causing food to get stuck between teeth. Food particles are the leading cause of cavities.

وقال صلى الله عليه وآله وسلم: القصعة تستغفر لمن يلحسها .

The Prophet ﷺ said, "The *qaṣʿa* (a type of bowl) seeks forgiveness for one who licks it."

Angels, animals, and in this case, even inanimate objects seek forgiveness for believers who are performing righteous deeds. This report encourages the adherent to avoid wastefulness.

The *qaṣ'a* is specifically mentioned, and it is a bowl that is made of wood. Research found that wooden utensils, cutting boards and plates have anti-bacterial qualities, while plastic surfaces enable disease-causing bacteria to persist.[13]

---

[13] Dean Cliver, "Cutting Boards of Plastic and Wood Contaminated Experimentally with Bacteria", Journal of Food Protection, https://jfoodprotection.org/doi/pdf/10.4315/0362-028X-57.1.16

Carbohydrates

❀ ❀ ❀

وقال صلى الله عليه وآله وسلم : خير طعامكم الخبز ، وخير فاكهتكم

العنب .

The Prophet 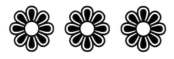 said, "The best of your foods is bread, and the best of your fruits is grapes."

Bread is a symbol of sustenance and blessing in the Judeo-Christian tradition. It has been a staple food for civilizations for thousands of years. Carbohydrates are the primary nutrient in bread, providing fuel to the body. However, pre-sliced white bread is made from a processed simple carbohydrate, which lacks fibre, loses nutrients, and can lead to obesity, diabetes, and heart disease.

Whole grain bread however is rich in vitamins and nutrients, and can reduce the risk of diabetes, heart disease, obesity, hypertension, and colon cancer.[14] In this tradition, the Prophet is giving bread hyperbolic emphasis due to its potential benefits.

Grapes are high in vitamin C and K. Grapes are very high in a number of powerful antioxidant compounds, which can prevent chronic illnesses: in fact, over 1,600 beneficial plant compounds have been identified in this fruit, especially in its skin and its seeds.[15] According to some studies, grapes may lower blood pressure, decrease cholesterol absorption, decrease blood sugar levels (due to the resveratrol in its skin)[16], improve retinal function, benefit brain health, and protect against bacteria, viruses, and yeast infections.[17]

وقال صلى الله عليه وآله وسلم : عليكم بالهريسة فأنها تنشط للعبادة

اربعين يوماً وهي التي انزلت علينا بدل مائدة عيسى عليه السلام .

The Prophet ﷺ said, "Betake to *harīsa* (a dish of meat and bulgur), for surely it encourages worship for forty days. It is what has been sent to us as a

[14] Megan Ware, "Is bread healthful or should I avoid it?", Medical News Today, https://www.medicalnewstoday.com/articles/295235
[15] Melissa Groves, "Top 12 Health Benefits of Eating Grapes", Healthline, https://www.healthline.com/nutrition/benefits-of-grapes#section1
[16] Kursvietene et al, "Multiplicity of effects and health benefits of resveratrol", US National Library of Medicine. https://www.ncbi.nlm.nih.gov/pubmed/27496184
[17] Melissa Groves, "Top 12 Health Benefits of Eating Grapes", Healthline, https://www.healthline.com/nutrition/benefits-of-grapes#section1

replacement of the table spread of Jesus, peace be upon him.”

The table spread of Jesus was sent by God from heaven to the apostles (5:112-115). The Christian communion, a practice based on this "last supper", traditionally uses bread. The above narration appears to share the idea that bulgur (another wheat) is a source of sustenance and blessing – one bestowed upon the Muslims as a replacement for what was given to the apostles. It would make sense therefore that the replacement would be better than that which came before it.

Bulgur is a common replacement for rice and other refined carbohydrates, because it is a better source of vitamins, minerals, fibre, and antioxidants. Bulgur is low in fat and high in minerals like magnesium and iron. Unlike most wheat flours, bulgur is not stripped of its bran and germ, which are where many nutrients are stored within a whole grain. Bulgur is both lower in calories and higher in fibre than quinoa. As a result of all of this, bulgur lowers the risk of cardiovascular disease and improves digestion.[18] Organic bulgur is sustainable, cruelty-free, and it has a low water and carbon footprint.

Mixed with the benefits of the protein in meat, bulgur will prepare one for longer and more frequent worship.

---

[18] Jillian Levy, "Bulgur Wheat: The Better Wheat for your Belly & More", Dr. Axe, https://draxe.com/nutrition/bulgur-wheat/

وقال صلى الله عليه وآله وسلم : الارز في الاطعمة كالسيد في القوم

وانا في الانبياء كالملح في الطعام .

The Prophet ﷺ said, "Rice is to food as the master is to the people, and I am to the prophets as salt is to food."

Rice is a staple dish in most cultures, as it is known to provide energy, minerals, and fibre, and help the body prevent illnesses.

The statement "I am to the prophets as salt is to food" may be a reference to the practice of starting and ending each meal with salt, as Muhammad ﷺ was the first prophet to be created and the last to be sent. It may further be a reference to Muhammad ﷺ preserving the message of the prophets. Lastly, it may be a reference to him being the "finishing touch" to the prophetic tradition after it was gradually built from Adam onward.

Water

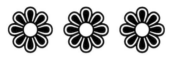

وقال صلى الله عليه وآله وسلم : سيد الاشربة في الدنيا والآخرة الماء.

The Prophet ﷺ said, "The master of drinks in this world and the Hereafter is water."

Allah says in the Quran, "And We have made from water every living thing." (21:30)

Water has the taste of life itself. It maintains the balance of bodily fluids, prevents dryness in the skin, helps your kidneys, and eases digestion.[19] Our bodies are made up of about 60% water, and thus water is needed for nutrient transportation and absorption, circulation, the

---

[19] James McIntosh, "Fifteen benefits of drinking water", Medical News Today, https://www.medicalnewstoday.com/articles/290814

creation of saliva, and the maintenance of a healthy body temperature.[20]

Water is to be drunk in three sips, and it is to be drunk whilst sitting.

The water of al-Kawthar in the Hereafter will flow from beneath the Throne of Allah. It will be whiter than milk and sweeter than honey. Those who drink from it will never be thirsty again.

وقال صلى الله عليه وآله وسلم : إن الحمى من قيح جهنم .

The Prophet ﷺ said, "Surely, fever is from the pus of Hell."

Fever is either a manifestation or a representation of hellfire in this world. In some traditions, fever is said to purify one from their sins. Every ache and pain that a believer experiences in this world is a trial and an atonement.

Just as water puts out fire, it is recommended to drink water during a fever. Fevers cause patients to sweat, and dehydration can worsen their symptoms and discomfort.

وقال صلى الله عليه وآله وسلم : إذا اشتهيتم الماء فاشربوه مصاً ، ولا تشربوه عباً .

---

[20] Ibid.

The Prophet ﷺ said, "If you should desire water, then drink it by sipping, and do not drink it by gulping."

Dr. Leonard Smith, a gastrointestinal, vascular and general surgeon advises, "If you drink too fast, you risk diluting your blood, which may cause faster excretion of water by the kidneys."[21] Thus, drinking water too quickly will cause your body to expel most of it as urine, which will slow down the hydration process.

وقال صلى الله عليه وآله وسلم : العب يورث الكباد .

The Prophet ﷺ said, "Gulping brings about *kubād* (ailment of the liver)."

This may be a reference to the iron levels in well water. As rain falls and seeps through iron-bearing soil and rock, iron can be dissolved into the water. Iron overload can be harmful to the liver, and it is common in patients with chronic liver disease.[22] However, iron deficiency

---

[21] Andrew Fiouzi, "If You're Chugging Water to Hydrate, You're Doing it Wrong", Mel Magazine, https://melmagazine.com/en-us/story/if-youre-chugging-water-to-hydrate-youre-doing-it-wrong

[22] Kowdley, "Iron Overload in Patients with Chronic Liver Disease", US National Library of Medicine, https://www.ncbi.nlm.nih.gov/pmc/articles/PMC5193089/

was the norm for most of human history, and so this *ḥadīth* may be a reference to another potential ailment.

Meat

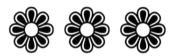

وقال صلى الله عليه وآله وسلم : ان ابليس يخطب شياطينه ويقول

عليكم باللحم ، والمسكر ، والناي ، فاني لا اجد جماع الشر إلا

فيها .

**The Prophet ﷺ said, "Surely, Iblīs exhorts his
devils, saying, 'Betake you to meat, intoxicants, and
the _nay_ (a type of flute), for surely I have not found
the aggregate of evil but in them."**

Eating meat is a _sunna_ of the Prophet, and the sacrifice
of an animal is an important aspect of Hajj. This is one
of the few traditions that speaks about the consumption
of meat in a negative way. While vegetarianism is not
recommended in Islam, one should not insist on eating
meat with every meal. It goes without saying that a

Muslim should not be tempted by any meat that is *ḥarām*.

There is no extant tradition of the Prophet eating beef. In one *ḥadīth*, the Prophet tells a man to not employ his son as a butcher, because "a butcher slaughters until mercy leaves his heart."[23] In a tradition attributed to Ali, he says, "Do not make your stomachs a graveyard of animals."[24]

In this *ḥadīth*, meat is grouped with intoxicants and flutes, perhaps due to its addictive and decadent qualities. The fleeting pleasure of these items can cause one to become heedless and distracted. The three are commonly enjoyed together in idle gatherings.

Studies have associated red meats with cardiovascular disease – this is especially true with processed red meats.[25]

وقال صلى الله عليه وآله وسلم : خير الادام في الدنيا والآخرة اللحم

.

---

[23] Tusi, *Tadhib al-Ahkam*, Volume 6, p. 362. https://bit.ly/2TJBSoz
[24] Ibn Abi'l Hadid, *Sharh Nahj al-Balagha*, http://islamport.com/w/lqh/Web/888/50.htm
[25] Mingyang Song et al, "Association of Animal and Plant Protein Intake With All-Cause and Cause-Specific Mortality." JAMA Internal Medicine, https://jamanetwork.com/journals/jamainternalmedicine/article-abstract/2540540

وقال صلى الله عليه وآله وسلم : اللحم ينبت اللحم ، ومن ترك اللحم

اربعين صباحاً ساء خلقه .

The Prophet ﷺ said, "The best condiment in this world and the Hereafter is meat.

Flesh grows flesh. One who gives up meat for forty days, his body is worsened."

It is no coincidence that most civilizations and even primitive societies consumed meat. Unlike plant-based sources of protein, red meats are packed with the same types of proteins that humans are made of, including myosin, actin, troponins, collagen, and other connective tissue proteins.[26] Red meats are also a major source of vitamin B12 and minerals. According to a 2004 study, conjugated linoleic acid, which is found in meat, can significantly reduce one's body fat mass.[27]

Regular red meat consumption can build and repeat tissues. A person on a high-protein diet is more likely to

---

[26] Robert Wildman, "Eat Your Meat: The Muscle-Building Bounty of Beef and Fish", Body Building,
https://www.bodybuilding.com/fun/eat-your-meat-the-muscle-building-bounty-of-beef-and-fish.html
[27] Gaullier JM et al, "Conjugated linoleic acid supplementation for 1 y reduces body fat mass in healthy overweight humans", US National Library of Medicine,
https://www.ncbi.nlm.nih.gov/pubmed/15159244

have a reduced appetite and a leaner body.[28] It boosts one's metabolism and increases fat burning.

White meats like chicken breast are high in protein and low in fat in comparison to red meat.

It is important to note that meat can be high in cholesterol, elevating one's risk of heart disease.[29] Some cuts of meat are lower in cholesterol – chicken breast is lower in cholesterol than chicken leg. Sirloin steak is lower in cholesterol than beef flank.[30]

"Flesh grows flesh", because protein is a building block for bones, muscles, cartilage, skin, and blood. One who avoids meat is "worsened", perhaps because it is difficult to maintain a fulfilling high-protein vegetarian diet, especially without access to proper supplements and alternatives.

وقال صلى الله عليه وآله وسلم : عليكم بأكل الجزور مخالفة لليهود.

The Prophet ﷺ said, "Betake you to the eating of the slaughtered camel, in contrast to the Jews."

---

[28] Halton TL et al, "The effects of high protein diets on thermogenesis, satiety and weight loss: a critical review", US National Library of Medicine, https://www.ncbi.nlm.nih.gov/pubmed/15466943
[29] Brian Krans, "Cholesterol Control: Chicken vs. Beef", Healthline, https://www.healthline.com/health/high-cholesterol/chicken-vs-beef#1
[30] Ibid.

When the Prophet established his state in Medina, the Jewish tribes wavered in their devotion to his leadership. 4:137 of the Quran shows an unstable environment, where the tribes believed in him one moment and disbelieved in him in the next. Hence, some Islamic laws were defined to distinguish those who followed the Prophet from those who did not. Leviticus 11:3-8 prohibits eating camel meat. According to some, one must renew their ablution after eating camel meat.

Camel meat has many medicinal functions, especially for those living in arid climates. It is a remedy for ailments such as seasonal fever, sciatica, shoulder pain, and asthma.[31] Camel meat is leaner than other meats and reduces the risk of cardiovascular disease. It has higher levels of calcium, minerals, and amino acids than beef.[32]

وقال صلى الله عليه وآله وسلم : من اكل اللحم اربعين يوماً صباحاً قسا قلبه .

The Prophet ﷺ said, "One who eats meats in the morning for forty days, his heart shall harden."

---

[31] Askale Abrhaley et al, "Medicinal value of camel milk and meat", Taylor & Francis Online, https://www.tandfonline.com/doi/full/10.1080/09712119.2017.13575 62

[32] Ibid.

There are at least two possible interpretations to this *ḥadīth*. Normally, a "hard heart" is an unkind, inhuman, apathetic, and numb state. Hard-heartedness is the root of all evil in Islamic spirituality. The goal is to maintain humility, sympathy, and selflessness toward our surroundings. The decadence of eating meat in the morning for forty days may make a person complacent, indulgent, and perhaps even careless about animals.

Another possible interpretation is that too much meat can lead to heart failure. In 2018, Dr. Jyrki Virtanen and other researchers released a study claiming that animal protein consumption can increase the risk of heart failure in middle-aged men.[33] However, Dr. Gregg Fonarow, a professor of cardiology at the University of California Los Angeles argues that this correlation may be due to other variables.[34]

وقال صلى الله عليه وآله وسلم : الشاة بركة ، والشاتان بركتان ،

وثلاث شياه غنيمة .

The Prophet ﷺ said, "A sheep is a blessing, two sheep are two blessings, and three sheep are *ghanīma* (profit, booty)."

---

[33] Heli E.K. Virtanen et al, "Intake of Different Dietary Proteins and Risk of Heart Failure in Men", US National Library of Medicine, https://www.ncbi.nlm.nih.gov/pmc/articles/PMC6023591/
[34] Steven Reinberg, "Too Much Meat, Dairy Tied to Heart Failure Risk", WebMD, https://www.webmd.com/heart-disease/heart-failure/news/20180529/too-much-meat-dairy-tied-to-heart-failure-risk#1

In pre-modern times, lamb was the red meat of choice in the Near East, not beef. Although lamb is higher in fat, lamb is a better source of vitamin K and vitamin D.[35] Lamb is also easier on the digestive tract than beef.

وقال صلى الله عليه وآله وسلم : لحم البقر داء ولبنها دواء ، ولحم الغنم دواء ولبنها داء .

The Prophet ﷺ said, "The meat of the cow is a malady, and its milk is a cure. The meat of the sheep is a cure, and its milk is a malady."

The benefits of choosing lamb over beef have been discussed earlier.

Despite some of the benefits of sheep's milk, it is higher in cholesterol and saturated fats than cow's milk, which can cause weight gain or even heart disease.[36]

---

[35] Ankita Lahon, "Lamb vs Beef: Difference in Nutritional Value, Health Benefits, and Taste", Foods for Better Health, https://www.foodsforbetterhealth.com/lamb-vs-beef-32858
[36] https://nutritiondata.self.com/facts/dairy-and-egg-products/94/2

Milk and Dairy

❀ ❀ ❀

وقال صلى الله عليه وآله وسلم : اسقوا نساءكم الحوامل الالبان فانها

تزيد في عقل الصبي .

The Prophet 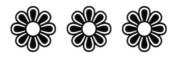 said, "Give your pregnant women milk to drink, for surely, it increases the intellect of the child."

A word of caution must be made that many people are lactose-intolerant or lactose-sensitive. In such cases, one should be aware of the symptoms and treatments of such conditions and take the necessary precautions.

A 2013 study published in the British Journal of Nutrition found that pregnant women who consumed lower amounts of iodine, which is found in milk, were more likely to have children with lower IQ scores and reading abilities.[37] Iodine is essential for producing hormones made by the thyroid gland, which has a direct effect on the development of the foetal brain. The researchers recommended that pregnant women consume milk, dairy products, and fish.

وقال صلى الله عليه وآله وسلم : إذا شربتم اللبن فتمضمضوا فان فيه دسماً .

The Prophet ﷺ said, "When you have drunken milk, wash your mouth, for surely there is fat in it."

The calcium in milk is good for dental hygiene, but one should wash their mouth or brush their teeth after drinking milk. Lactose and sugar that remains on your teeth overnight can cause cavities and tooth decay.[38]

Tooth decay is the single most common chronic childhood illness worldwide.[39] It is thus important to

---

[37] Claire Carter, "Drink milk to increase child's IQ, pregnant women told", The Telegraph, https://www.telegraph.co.uk/news/health/news/10072366/Drink-milk-to-increase-childs-IQ-pregnant-women-told.html

[38] "How milk affects your teeth", Pompton Lakes Dentistry, https://www.pomptonlakesdentistry.com/how-milk-affects-your-teeth.html

[39] Sujata Tungare et al, "Baby Bottle Syndrome", US National Library of Medicine, https://www.ncbi.nlm.nih.gov/books/NBK535349/

encourage new mothers to be aware of the cavities that bottled milk or even breastmilk can cause.[40]

وقال صلى الله عليه وآله وسلم : ثلاثة لا ترد ، الوسادة ، واللبن ، والدهن.

The Prophet ﷺ said, "Do not decline three: the cushion, milk, and oil."

Along with mattresses, pillows play an important role in supporting healthy spinal alignment during sleep. The healthiest sleeping position is one's right side, which is supported in the Sunna. Those who sleep on their sides need a pillow to work in conjunction with their mattress to keep their spine straight while they sleep. Otherwise, the weight of their head will wrench their neck downwards and out of alignment with the rest of their spine. Sleeping on your shoulder puts undue pressure on your shoulder and arm muscles.

Milk provides potassium, B12, calcium, and vitamin D, which are lacking in many diets.[41] It is also a good source

---

[40] Von Burg MM et al, "Baby bottle tooth decay: a concern for all mothers", US National Library of Medicine, https://www.ncbi.nlm.nih.gov/pubmed/8700605

[41] Murphy SP, "Child and Adult Care Food Program: Aligning Dietary Guidance for All", US National Library of Medicine, https://www.ncbi.nlm.nih.gov/books/NBK209825/

of protein, vitamin A, magnesium, zinc, thiamine, and omega 3.

The reference to oil is probably a reference to skincare. Olive oil, for example, fights off cancer-causing cells for those exposed to UV rays.[42] Olive oil is an antioxidant that is rich in vitamins and fights off bacteria.[43]

وقال صلى الله عليه وآله وسلم : أكل الجبن داء ، والجوز دواء ، فاذا اجتمعا معاً صارا دواءاً .

The Prophet ﷺ said, "Eating cheese is a malady, and the walnut is a remedy. So, if they are brought together, then they become a remedy."

Calcium alone cannot build strong bones and tissues. Research shows calcium needs phosphorus to maximize its bone-strengthening benefits.[44] This is especially important for those suffering from osteoporosis. Whilst

---

[42] Arief Budiyanto et al, "Protective effect of topically applied olive oil against photocarcinogenesis following UVB exposure of mice", Oxford Academic, https://academic.oup.com/carcin/article/21/11/2085/2908770

[43] "Olive Oil Benefits for Your Face", Healthline, https://www.healthline.com/health/olive-oil-benefits-face

[44] Michael A. Friedman et al, "Calcium- and Phosphorus-Supplemented Diet Increases Bone Mass after Short-Term Exercise and Increases Bone Mass and Structural Strength after Long-Term Exercise in Adult Mice", US National Library of Medicine, https://www.ncbi.nlm.nih.gov/pmc/articles/PMC4805202/

cheese also contains phosphorus, walnuts are high in phosphorus.

وقال صلى الله عليه وآله وسلم : عليكم بالألبان فانها تمسح الحر عن القلب كما يكسح الاصبع العرق عن الجبين ، وتشد الظهر وتزيد في العقل وتذكي الذهن وتجلو البصر وتذهب النسيان .

The Prophet ﷺ said, "Betake you to milk, for it wipes heat from the heart as the fingers sweep sweat from the forehead. It strengthens the back, increases the intellect, kindles the mind, clarifies vision, and removes forgetfulness."

If this narration is referring to heartburn, then some have noted that the calcium and protein content in milk can be helpful in treating acid reflux. However, the fat in milk can potentially make heartburn worse.[45]

While there is no scientific consensus on the affect of milk on the heart, according to a 2017 aggregate study, dairy consumption was associated with a 10% lower risk of cardiovascular disease and a 12% lower risk of

---

[45] Ariane Lang, "Does Milk Relieve Heartburn?", Healthline, https://www.healthline.com/nutrition/milk-for-heartburn

stroke.[46] This is further corroborated by other acclaimed studies.[47] [48]

The calcium in milk would surely strengthen one's bones and therefore one's back.

According to a study at the University of Kansas conducted by Dr. Debra Sullivan, participants who drink milk regularly have higher levels of glutathione in their brains.[49] Glutathione helps stave off oxidative stress, and reduces the risk of Alzheimer's, Parkinson's, and many other conditions.

Milk is a good source of riboflavin and can help reduce your risk of cataracts. The vitamin A in milk is also a leading performer among eye health vitamins.[50]

---

[46] Fatemah Gholami et al, "The effect of dairy consumption on the prevention of cardiovascular diseases: A meta-analysis of prospective studies", US National Library of Medicine, https://www.ncbi.nlm.nih.gov/pmc/articles/PMC5402021/

[47] Alexander DD et al, "Dairy consumption and CVD: a systematic review and meta-analysis", US National Library of Medicine, https://www.ncbi.nlm.nih.gov/pubmed/26786887

[48] Drouin-Chartier JP et al, "Systematic Review of the Association between Dairy Product Consumption and Risk of Cardiovascular-related Clinical Outcomes", US National Library of Medicine, https://www.ncbi.nlm.nih.gov/pubmed/28140321

[49] Andy Hyland, "Drinking Milk May Be Good For Your Brain", Futurity, https://www.futurity.org/milk-glutathione-879052/

[50] Holley Grainger, "Healthy food for your eyes", CNN, https://www.cnn.com/2010/HEALTH/04/17/eyes.healthy.eating.foods/index.html

A 2014 study showed that greater milk and dairy intake reduced the risk of dementia among a sample of the elderly in Japan.[51]

وقال صلى الله عليه وآله وسلم : ليس يجزي مكان الطعام والشراب غير اللبن .

The Prophet ﷺ said, "Nothing takes the place of food and drink except for milk."

Milk can be a good substitute to some meals. Milk is rich in calcium, potassium, vitamin B12, vitamin D, protein, and choline; making it essential for healthy bones and teeth, reduced blood pressure, a regulated mood and sleep pattern, and muscle-building.[52] Drinking milk can help control portion size and therefore calorie intake, while providing casein and calcium and decreasing fat deposits in the blood.

---

[51] Ozawa M et al, "Milk and dairy consumption and risk of dementia in an elderly Japanese population: the Hisayama Study", US National Library of Medicine,
https://www.ncbi.nlm.nih.gov/pubmed/24916840
[52] Megan Ware, "All about milk", Medical News Today,
https://www.medicalnewstoday.com/articles/273451#health_benefit s_of_milk

Honey

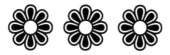

وقال صلى الله عليه وآله وسلم : ثلاثة يفرح بهن الجسم ويربو ،
الطيب ولباس اللين ، وشرب العسل .

The Prophet ﷺ said, "There are three that delight the body and sustain it: perfume, soft clothing, and drinking honey."

Perfume has been shown to improve moods and regulate heart rates.[53]

Cotton fabric is breathable and transmits moisture away from one's skin. Cotton clothing protects against from heat in the summer and cold in the winter by providing thermal insulation as the cotton fabric traps air between

---

[53] Rachel Herz, "Neurobiology of Sensation and Reward", US National Library of Medicine, https://www.ncbi.nlm.nih.gov/books/NBK92802/

the fabric fibres. Cotton also rarely causes allergic reactions and is hypoallergenic. It is soft, stretchable, and comfortable.

Honey is a popular item in Islamic medicine. It is rich in antioxidants,[54] which are linked to a reduced risk of heart attacks and some forms of cancer. Honey reduces total and "bad" cholesterol while significantly raising "good" cholesterol.[55] A review of 26 studies on honey and wound care found honey most effective at healing partial-thickness burns and wounds that have become infected after surgery.[56] Honey alleviates allergies by soothing and reducing coughing.[57] A 2011 study showed that the immediate memory of healthy postmenopausal women improved after sixteen weeks of taking a honey supplement.[58]

---

[54] Gheldof N, "Identification and quantification of antioxidant components of honeys from various floral sources", US National Library of Medicine,
https://www.ncbi.nlm.nih.gov/pubmed/12358452

[55] Yaghoobi N, "Natural honey and cardiovascular risk factors; effects on blood glucose, cholesterol, triacylglycerol, CRP, and body weight compared with sucrose", US National Library of Medicine,
https://www.ncbi.nlm.nih.gov/pubmed/18454257

[56] Jull AB, "Honey as a topical treatment for wounds", US National Library of Medicine,
https://www.ncbi.nlm.nih.gov/pubmed/25742878

[57] Lizette Borreli, "Liquid Gold: 7 Health Benefits of Honey That Could Heal Your Whole Body", Medical Daily,
https://www.medicaldaily.com/liquid-gold-7-health-benefits-honey-could-heal-your-whole-body-325932

[58] Zahiruddin Othman, "Improvement in immediate memory after 16 weeks of tualang honey (Agro Mas) supplement in healthy postmenopausal women", Menopause,
https://www.academia.edu/3228620/Improvement_in_immediate_m

وقال صلى الله عليه وآله وسلم : نعم الشراب العسل يربي ويذهب

درن الصدر .

The Prophet ﷺ said, "The most excellent drink is honey. It sustains [the body] and removes filth (or tuberculosis) from the chest."

The affect of honey on tuberculosis is a subject that has not been thoroughly studied. Tuberculosis is most prevalent in Sub-Saharan Africa, and a study done in Uganda suggests that honey inhibits tuberculosis bacteria and quickens the healing process.[59] This may be because honey reduces inflammation in the bronchial tubes, helps break up mucus, and suppresses coughing.[60]

Tuberculosis is an aggressive bacterium that usually requires antibiotics. Honey can aid in boosting one's immunity, but it is not necessarily an end-all-be-all solution to the illness.

emory_after_16_weeks_of_tualang_honey_Agro_Mas_supplement_in _healthy_postmenopausal_women

[59] Brain Ssenoga, "Honey can treat TB – researchers", The Observer, https://www.observer.ug/news-headlines/41473-honey-can-treat-tb-researchers

[60] James Roland, "Honey for Asthma: Can Honey Treat Asthma?", Healthline, https://www.healthline.com/health/asthma/honey-for-asthma

Dates

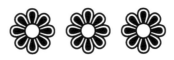

وقال صلى الله عليه وآله وسلم : إذا ولدت المرأة فليكن اول ما تأكل الرطب الحلو والتمر فأنه لو كان شيء افضل منه اطعمه الله تعالى مريم حين ولدت عيسى عليه السلام .

The Prophet ﷺ said, "When a woman gives birth, then let the first thing she eats be sweet fresh dates and dried ones, for if there were a thing better than it, Allah the Exalted would have fed it to Mary when she gave birth to Jesus, peace be upon him."

When Mary was suffering the pangs of labour, a voice called, "Do not grieve, for your Lord has provided beneath you a stream. Shake toward you the trunk of the palm tree; it will drop upon you ripe, fresh dates. So, eat and drink and be contented." (19:24-25) Thus, the

Quran presents dates as a treatment for women in labour.

A 2017 controlled study found that women who consumed dates during late pregnancy and the onset of labour had significantly less need for labour augmentation.[61] Dates have an oxytocin-like effect on the body, leading to increased sensitivity of the uterus; they also stimulate uterine contractions and reduce postpartum hemorrhage.[62] A 2011 study found that women who ate six dates a day for the four weeks leading up to their due date were 74% more dilated than women who didn't eat dates.[63]

وقال صلى الله عليه وآله وسلم : كل التمر على الريق فانه يقتل الدود.

The Prophet ﷺ said, "Eat the date on an empty stomach, for it kills the worm."

Garlic, onions, coconuts, figs, dates, chicory, avocado seeds, ginger, black pepper and pomegranates are examples of foods shown to promote antiparasitic

[61] Razali N et al, "Date fruit consumption at term: Effect on length of gestation, labour and delivery", US National Library of Medicine, https://www.ncbi.nlm.nih.gov/pubmed/28286995
[62] Masoumeh Kordi et al, "The Effect of Late Pregnancy Consumption of Date Fruit on Cervical Ripening in Nulliparous Women", Journal of Midwifery and Reproductive Health, http://jmrh.mums.ac.ir/article_2772_0.html
[63] Al-Kuran et al, "The effect of late pregnancy consumption of date fruit on labour and delivery", US National Library of Medicine, https://www.ncbi.nlm.nih.gov/pubmed/21280989

activity in laboratory or animal studies, but the effectiveness of these foods has not yet been properly evaluated in humans.[64]

وقال صلى الله عليه وآله وسلم : نعم السحور للمؤمن التمر .

The Prophet ﷺ said, "The date is an excellent *suḥūr* for the believer."

It is reported that the Prophet said, "When the growing season for dates comes, then congratulate me; and when it goes, then console me." (وقال صلى الله عليه وآله وسلم : إذا

جاء الرطب فهنئوني ، وإذا ذهب فعزوني .)

The relationship between the Prophet and the date may be that they are both sweet, nourishing things that came out of an arid, hostile environment.

Suḥūr is a practice that was established to distinguish the Muslims from Jewish fasting. However, *suḥūr* is also a great way to get through a long fast. Dates are high in fibre, which helps a person feel full for longer.[65] Dates are high in antioxidants that can protect the body from inflammation. They are also a source of potassium,

---

[64] Reem Ibrahim, "Can Certain Foods Kill Intestinal Parasites?", Healthfully, https://healthfully.com/kill-parasites-activated-charcoal-6746476.html
[65] Rachel Nall, "Are dates healthful?", Medical News Today, https://www.medicalnewstoday.com/articles/322548

which is good for cardiovascular health,[66] as it reduces blood pressure.

وقال صلى الله عليه وآله وسلم : من وجد التمر فليفطر عليه ، ومن لم يجد فليفطر على الماء فانه طهور .

The Prophet ﷺ said, "One who finds a date, then he is to break his fast with it; and one who does not come upon one, then he is to break his fast with water, for surely it is a purifier."

According to Swati Kapoor, a dietician and nutritionist, there are several benefits to drinking water on an empty stomach. It cleanses the colon, increasing the efficiency of the intestine to absorb nutrients; it helps in correcting bowel movement, and it increases the body's efficiency in fighting infections.[67]

---

[66] Ibid.
[67] Swati Kapoor, "5 Benefits of Drinking Water on an Empty Stomach", Practo, https://www.practo.com/healthfeed/5-benefits-of-drinking-water-on-an-empty-stomach-4931/post

Fruits

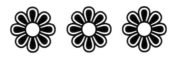

وقال صلى الله عليه وآله وسلم : اكل التين امان من القولنج .

The Prophet ﷺ said, "Eating figs is a protection against colic."

Infantile colic refers to long episodes of crying in children. Colic does not typically have long-term effects on the children, but it can lead to postpartum depression in parents and even abuse towards the child.

In a *ḥadīth* attributed to the Prophet, he said, "Do not beat your children when they cry, for four months of their crying is their witnessing that there is no god but Allah, four months blessing the Prophet, and four months praying for their parents." (لا تضربوا أطفالكم على بكائهم فان

بكاءهم أربعة أشهر شهادة ان لا إله إلا الله، وأربعة أشهر الصلاة على النبي
(صلى الله عليه وآله، و أربعة الدعاء لوالديه

The cause of colic is not fully known, but it may be caused by the mother's diet. Specifically, the consumption of dairy is a culprit.[68] [69] If this is the case, then figs are an excellent alternative source of calcium – figs have more calcium than other dried fruits.[70]

وقال صلى الله عليه وآله وسلم : كل التين فانه ينفع البواسير والنقرس.

The Prophet ﷺ said, "Eat figs, for they help with hemorrhoids and gout."

Figs are a proven remedy against constipation, which is a cause of hemorrhoids. Whether they are eaten fresh or dried, they naturally exert a laxative effect.[71]

There is insufficient available research on the affect of figs on gout.

---

[68] Adam Felman, "Everything you need to know about colic", Medical News Today, https://www.medicalnewstoday.com/articles/162806

[69] "Diet-Related Colic: When to Suspect It and What to Do", Bellamy's Organic, https://www.bellamysorganic.com.au/blog/diet-related-colic-when-to-suspect-it-and-what-to-do/

[70] Kerri-Ann Jennings, "Top 15 Calcium-Rich Foods (Many Are Non-Dairy)", Healthline, https://www.healthline.com/nutrition/15-calcium-rich-foods

[71] Ashley K. Willington, *Natural Hemorrhoids Remedies: How to Get Rid of Hemorrhoids Forever*, Chapter 1.

وقال صلى الله عليه وآله وسلم : اكل السفرجل يذهب ظلمة البصر.

The Prophet ﷺ said, "Eating quince removes the darkness of vision."

Quince is a fruit from the Rosaceae family that resembles apples and pears. Quince is reportedly used to soothe eye problems.[72] [73]

وقال صلى الله عليه وآله وسلم : ربيع امتي العنب والبطيخ .

The Prophet ﷺ said, "The springtime of my Umma is the grape and the melon."

Melons such as cantaloupes are a refreshing and healthful fruit. The fibre, potassium, vitamin C, and choline in cantaloupe all support heart health. A cup of cantaloupe provides 10% of one's recommended daily intake of potassium, which helps decrease blood pressure.[74] With its high water and electrolyte contents,

---

[72] "Quince", WebMD,
https://www.webmd.com/vitamins/ai/ingredientmono-384/quince
[73] Saba, "15 Amazing Health Benefits of Quince Fruit",
https://www.stylecraze.com/articles/amazing-health-benefits-of-quince-fruit/#12-treats-liver-and-eye-diseases
[74] Megan Ware, "Everything you need to know about cantaloupe", Medical News Today,
https://www.medicalnewstoday.com/articles/279176

cantaloupe boosts hydration after a hot day or a
workout.[75]

وعن ابن عباس انه قال صلى الله عليه وآله : عليكم بالبطيخ فان فيه
عشر خصال هو طعام وشراب واسنان وريحان يغسل المثانة ويغسل
البطن ويكثر ماء الظهر ويزيد في الجماع ويقطع البرودة وينقي البشرة.

**"From Ibn ʿAbbās that he ﷺ said: Betake you to
the melon, for in it are ten traits: it is food, drink, [it
is good for the] teeth, it has a good smell, it washes
the bladder and washes the stomach, it increases
the water of the back, it increases one in sexual
intercourse, it breaks coldness, and it cleanses the
skin."**

Melons have high water content and provide fibre.[76]
Fibre and water can help prevent constipation,
promoting a healthy digestive tract.

Melons are also a good source of vitamin A, which
contributes to the growth and maintenance of skin and
muscle tissues. They are also high in vitamin C, which
enables the body to produce collagen.[77]

Watermelon may be an aphrodisiac, as it is rich in
citrulline, an amino acid that relaxes and dilates blood

---

[75] Ibid.
[76] Ibid.
[77] Ibid.

vessels. This may make watermelons a good treatment for erectile disfunction.[78]

وقال صلى الله عليه وآله وسلم : عليكم بالرمان وكلوا شحمه فانه دباغ المعدة وما من حبة تقع في جوف احدكم إلا انارت قلبه وحبسته من الشيطان والوسوسة اربعين يوماً .

The Prophet ﷺ said, "Betake you to the pomegranate and eat its pulp for it is the tanner (i.e. softener) of the stomach. There is not a seed that enters the mouth of one of you but that it illuminates his heart and holds back from Satan and the whispering (al-waswasa, i.e. of the Devil) for forty days."

Waswasa refers to irrational doubts in Islamic rituals, especially ablution and prayer. There are a couple of reports that associate the eating of pomegranates with keeping Satan or *waswās* away. However, one may still be subject to the habits of their *nafs*.

Pomegranate benefits your digestive system by providing B-complex vitamins that help your body efficiently convert fat, protein and carbohydrates into energy. One fruit provides 25% of the folate and about one sixth of the thiamin, riboflavin and vitamin B6 you need daily. It also provides 11 grams of fibre, more than twice the

---

[78] Zawn Villines, "Can watermelon help with erectile disfunction?", Medical News Today, https://www.medicalnewstoday.com/articles/320440

amount of fibre in a bowl of bran flakes.[79] Fibre helps food move through your body effectively, assisting with digestion.

Pomegranate is also a rich source of antioxidants that limit the formation of fatty plaques in the arteries.[80]

وقال صلى الله عليه وآله وسلم : عليكم بالاترج فانه ينير الفوائد ويزيد في الدماغ .

The Prophet ﷺ said, "Betake you to citron, for surely, it illuminates the heart and adds to the brain."

A study published in the Journal of Epidemiology showed that frequent consumption of citrus fruits was associated with a lower risk of heart disease and stroke among 10,623 people.[81] A 2017 study had similar findings, reporting that a higher intake of citrus fruits

[79] Gabriel Cousens, "Pomegranate and Digestion", Gabriel Cousens MD, http://treeoflifecenterus.com/pomegranate-and-digestion/
[80] Michael Aviram et al, "Pomegranate for Your Cardiovascular Health", US National Library of Medicine, https://www.ncbi.nlm.nih.gov/pmc/articles/PMC3678830/
[81] Yamada T et al, "Frequency of citrus fruit intake is associated with the incidence of cardiovascular disease: the Jichi Medical School cohort study", US National Library of Medicine, https://www.ncbi.nlm.nih.gov/pubmed/21389640

was linked to a lower risk of heart disease and even death.[82]

Several studies in older adults have shown that citrus fruits may boost brain function.[83] [84] [85] The flavonoids in citrus fruits may also ward off neurodegenerative diseases, such as Alzheimer's and Parkinson's, which result from the breakdown of cells in the nervous system. These diseases, in part, are caused by inflammation; and flavonoids in citrus fruits have anti-inflammatory capabilities that help protect against the deterioration of the nervous system.[86] [87]

---

[82] Aune D et al, "Fruit and vegetable intake and the risk of cardiovascular disease, total cancer and all-cause mortality- a systematic review and dose-response meta-analysis of prospective studies.", US National Library of Medicine, https://www.ncbi.nlm.nih.gov/pubmed/28338764

[83] "Mudi H. Alharbi et al, "Flavonoid-rich orange juice is associated with acute improvements in cognitive function in healthy middle-aged males", US National Library of Medicine, https://www.ncbi.nlm.nih.gov/pmc/articles/PMC5009163/

[84] Nurk E et al, "Cognitive performance among the elderly in relation to the intake of plant foods. The Hordaland Health Study", US National Library of Medicine, https://www.ncbi.nlm.nih.gov/pubmed/20550741/

[85] Kean RJ et al, "Chronic consumption of flavanone-rich orange juice is associated with cognitive benefits: an 8-wk, randomized, double-blind, placebo-controlled trial in healthy older adults", US National Library of Medicine, https://www.ncbi.nlm.nih.gov/pubmed/25733635/

[86] Cirmi S, "Neurodegenerative Diseases: Might Citrus Flavonoids Play a Protective Role?", US National Library of Medicine, https://www.ncbi.nlm.nih.gov/pubmed/27706034

[87] Elumalai P et al, "Role of Quercetin Benefits in Neurodegeneration", US National Library of Medicine, https://www.ncbi.nlm.nih.gov/pubmed/27651256

وقال صلى الله عليه وآله وسلم : كل الباذنجان واكثر فانها شجرة

رأيتها في الجنة . فمن اكلها على انها داء كانت داءً ، ومن اكلها

على انها دواء كانت دواءً .

The Prophet ﷺ said, "Eat eggplant often, for it is a plant that I saw in Paradise. So, one who eats it thinking that it is a malady, then it is a malady; and one who eats it thinking that it is a remedy, then it is a remedy."

According to this report, eggplant is a fruit of Paradise that the Prophet may have seen during his ascension (mi' rāj). If it is paradisal, then it must in essence be good.

The narration appears to iterate the logic of placebo, as one who simply believes that the eggplant is harmful will be harmed, and one who simply believes that the eggplant is beneficial will find benefit. A common theory is that one's expectation can cause one's body to produce effects similar to what a medication might have caused, positive or negative.[88] The stronger the expectation, the stronger the effect. This shows the significance of one's mindset in healing – optimism has a biomedical function. In truth, healing is a very human experience, as humans are the only beings that are

---

[88] "What is the Placebo Effect?", WebMD, https://www.webmd.com/pain-management/what-is-the-placebo-effect#1

known to ingest a substance with the hope, faith, and knowledge that they will recover.

Eggplants are mostly beneficial to one's health. The fibre, potassium, vitamins, antioxidants, anthocyanins and flavonoids can reduce the risk of heart disease, decrease levels of bad cholesterol, reduce the risk of non-alcoholic fatty liver disease, help prevent tumor growth, and help prevent age-related macular degeneration in the eyes.[89]

وقال صلى الله عليه وآله وسلم : عليكم بالزبيب فانه يطفي المرة ويسكن البلغم ويشد العصب ويذهب النصب ويحسن القلب .

The Prophet ﷺ said, "Betake you to raisins, for they quench the bile, calm the phlegm, strengthen the nerve, get rid of fatigue, and ameliorate the heart."

A 2003 study found that daily consumption of sun-dried raisins significantly decreased fecal bile acids in healthy adults, which may decrease the risk of colon cancer.[90]

---

[89] Megan Ware, "Eggplant health benefits and tasty tips", Medical News Today, https://www.medicalnewstoday.com/articles/279359
[90] Spiller GA et al, "Effect of sun-dried raisins on bile acid excretion, intestinal transit time, and fecal weight: a dose-response study", US National Library of Medicine, https://www.ncbi.nlm.nih.gov/pubmed/12935318

The raisins in a 1.5-ounce box have 322 milligrams or 7 percent of the recommended daily intake of potassium.[91] Potassium is able to carry electrical charges that cause muscle contraction and stimulate nerve impulses.

The 34 grams of carbohydrates in one small box of raisins include 26 grams of sugar for rapid energy. One will also get 1.6 grams of fibre, which is 4 percent of men's and 6 percent of women's daily intake. About half of the total is soluble fibre that helps lower cholesterol and balance blood sugar.[92]

According to a study conducted at the American College of Cardiology, a routine consumption of raisins may significantly lower blood pressure.[93]

وقال صلى الله عليه وآله وسلم : العناب يذهب بالحمى والكحة ويجلي القلب .

The Prophet ﷺ said, "The jujube removes the fever and the cough, and clarifies the heart."

---

[91] Sandi Busch, "What Are the Benefits of Eating Raisins Everyday?", SFGate, https://healthyeating.sfgate.com/benefits-eating-raisins-day-5982.html

[92] Ibid.

[93] Beth Casteel, "Snacking on raisins may offer a heart-healthy way to lower blood pressure", American College of Cardiology, https://www.acc.org/about-acc/press-releases/2012/03/25/15/51/raisins_bp

A jujube is a small fruit that resembles a date and tastes like an apple. Jujubes. are used for various conditions including fever and lung disorders.[94]

Jujubes' antioxidant and anti-inflammatory abilities may deliver broad benefits and protections to the cardiovascular system.[95]

وقال صلى الله عليه وآله وسلم : ما من امرأة حاملة اكلت البطيخ إلا

يكون مولودها حسن الوجه والخلق .

The Prophet ﷺ said, "There is not a pregnant woman who eats melon but that her child shall be comely of face and form."

As long as a cantaloupe is washed thoroughly, it can safely be eaten during pregnancy. Cantaloupes support the growth of a fetus' heart, lungs, kidneys, eyes and bones. Being rich in vitamin A and folic acid, cantaloupe helps prevent neural tube defects. The calcium content

---

[94] Xinwen Jin, "Ziziphus jujube", Science Direct, https://www.sciencedirect.com/topics/agricultural-and-biological-sciences/jujube

[95] Souleymane Abdoul-Azize, "Potential Benefits of Jujube (Zizyphus Lotus L), Bioactive Compounds for Nutrition and Health", US National Library of Medicine, https://www.ncbi.nlm.nih.gov/pmc/articles/PMC5174181/

helps in the formation of healthy bone and tooth structures in the baby.[96]

Cantaloupes should not be considered an alternative to folic acid supplementation as recommended by a doctor.

[96] Rebecca Malachi, "Is It Safe To Eat Muskmelon During Pregnancy?", Mom Junction, https://www.momjunction.com/articles/is-it-safe-to-eat-muskmelon-during-pregnancy_0088031/#gref

Aromatic
Plants

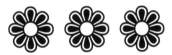

وقال صلى الله عليه وآله وسلم : شموا النرجس ولو في اليوم مرة ، ولو

في الاسبوع مرة ، ولو في الشهر مرة ، ولو في السنة مرة ، ولو في

الدهر مرة ، فان في القلب حبة من الجنون والجذام والبرص وشمه

يقلعها .

The Prophet ﷺ said, "Smell the narcissus, even if only once a day, and even if only once a week, and even if only once a month, and even if only once a year, and even if only once an epoch. For surely, in the heart is a seed of madness, leprosy, and vitiligo, and its smell weeds it out."

Aromatherapy is an age-old Islamic medicinal practice. Some reports indicate that perfumes have a paradisal origin and have healing qualities. The Prophet famously loved perfumes and had the scent of musk. Regarding Paradise, the Prophet said, "Its soil is white, shining, pure musk" (دَرْمَكَةٌ بَيْضَاءُ مِسْكٌ خَالِصٌ) and even "sweeter than musk" (أَطْيَبُ مِنَ الْمِسْكِ).

Galantamine is one of a number of alkaloids found in the daffodil family. It is used to treat dementia and early Alzheimer's, because it reduces the rate that acetylcholine is broken down in the brain. This helps brain cells communicate with each other more efficiently and is essential for memory and thought.[97]

Daffodils are used in traditional sub-Saharan African medicine to treat leprosy. However, there is insufficient research on its effects.

وقال صلى الله عليه وآله وسلم : الحناء خضاب الاسلام يزيد في المؤمن عمله ويذهب بالصداع ويحد البصر ويزيد في الوقاع وهو سيد الرياحين في الدنيا والآخرة .

The Prophet ﷺ said, "Henna is the dye of Islam. It increases the believer in his work, gets rid of headaches, limits vitiligo, and increases sexual

---

[97] "Galantamine", US National Library of Medicine, https://medlineplus.gov/druginfo/meds/a699058.html

intercourse. It is the master of aromatic plants (*rayaḥīn*) in this world and the Hereafter."

Henna is often used as a dye, scent, and adornment in the Muslim world.

The antioxidant activity in the roots of this plant are useful in the treatment of leprosy.[98] Henna is also used as a treatment for headaches;[99] though some report allergic reactions, and henna causing headaches due to its weight.

Henna has traditionally been used as an aphrodisiac and it is even mentioned in the Kama Sutra. The application of scents is a common sexual practice.

وقال صلى الله عليه وآله وسلم : ما من ورقة من ورق الهندباء إلا عليها قطرة من ماء الجنة .

The Prophet ﷺ said, "There is not a leaf from the endive (or chicory) leaves but that upon it is a drop from the water of Paradise."

Endive is a leafy green which is rich in fibre, thus supporting digestion. It is also loaded with antioxidants,

---

[98] Susi Endrini et al, "Anticarcinogenic Properties and Antioxidant Activity of Henna", Science Alert, https://scialert.net/fulltext/?doi=jms.2002.194.197
[99] "Henna", WebMD, https://www.webmd.com/vitamins/ai/ingredientmono-854/henna

including quercetin, kaempferol, myricetin and others. It is a great source of vitamin K, which strengthens bone health.[100] A 2016 study showed that endive extract reduced drug-induced liver damage in rats.[101]

وقال صلى الله عليه وآله وسلم : من اراد ان يريح فليشم الورد الاحمر.

The Prophet ﷺ said, "Whomever wishes to relax is to smell the red rose."

Rosewater has been used in several controlled studies to reduce anxiety in patients. A 2016 study showed that when hemodialysis patients inhaled rosewater for four weeks, their anxiety was noticeably reduced.[102] In a 2014 study, nulliparous women in the first stage of labour were given rose oil and footbaths, which reduced their anxiety significantly.[103]

---

[100] Rachael Link, "What is Endive Good For? Top 5 Benefits of This Leafy Green", Dr. Axe, https://draxe.com/nutrition/what-is-endive/
[101] Elgengaihi S et al, "Hepatoprotective Efficacy of Cichorium intybus L. Extract Against Carbon Tetrachloride-induced Liver Damage in Rats", US National Library of Medicine, https://www.ncbi.nlm.nih.gov/pubmed/26913368
[102] Barati F, "The Effect of Aromatherapy on Anxiety in Patients", US National Library of Medicine, https://www.ncbi.nlm.nih.gov/pubmed/27878109
[103] Kheirkhah M, "Comparing the effects of aromatherapy with rose oils and warm foot bath on anxiety in the first stage of labor in nulliparous women", US National Library of Medicine, https://www.ncbi.nlm.nih.gov/pubmed/?term=red+rose+aromatherapy

وقال صلى الله عليه وآله وسلم : الشونيز دواء من كل داء إلا السام.

The Prophet ﷺ **said, "***Shūnīz* **(black seed) is a cure for every malady except for death."**

Expressions like the one above are usually hyperbolic literary devices. This supplement does not necessarily replace medication, and in some cases, it can cause allergic reactions, constipation, vomiting, and adverse interactions with other medication.

Nonetheless, black seed oil has a wide range of benefits. A 2018 meta-analysis concluded that it exerts a moderate effect on the reduction of body weight.[104]

A controlled study in 2013 found that black seed oil had the same efficacy as Betamethasone (a steroid medication) in decreasing the severity of hand eczema.[105]

Research suggests that the antimicrobial and anti-inflammatory effects of black seed oil can improve acne. A 2015 study published by the Journal of Dermatology & Dermatologic Surgery found that 93% of participants reported moderate to good results.[106]

---

[104] Namazi N et al, "The effects of Nigella sativa L. on obesity: A systematic review and meta-analysis", US National Library of Medicine, https://www.ncbi.nlm.nih.gov/pubmed/?term=The+effects+of+Nigella+sativa+L.+on+obesity%3A+A+systematic+review+and+meta-analysis

[105] Yousefi M, "Comparison of therapeutic effect of topical Nigella with Betamethasone and Eucerin in hand eczema", US National Library of Medicine. https://www.ncbi.nlm.nih.gov/pubmed/23198836

[106] Salih H.M. Aljabre et al, "Dermatological effects of Nigella sativa", Science Direct,

The thymoquinone in black seed oil can influence programmed cell death, or apoptosis, in several types of cancer cell. These include brain cancer,[107] leukemia,[108] and breast cancer cells.[109]

A 2013 controlled study showed that black seed oil reduced kidney and liver disease in rats.[110] Its effect on human kidney and livers however is still not known.

According to an article published by the Journal of Endocrinology & Metabolism, black seed oil may have antidiabetic properties and improve blood sugar levels.[111] Again, this study used animal models, so more research is necessary to confirm the effectiveness of the oil in humans.

https://www.sciencedirect.com/science/article/pii/S23522410150002 86

[107] Ira O. Racoma et al, "Thymoquinone Inhibits Autophagy and Induces Cathepsin-Mediated, Caspase-Independent Cell Death in Glioblastoma Cells", US National Library of Medicine, https://www.ncbi.nlm.nih.gov/pmc/articles/PMC3767730/

[108] Landa Zeenalabdin Ali Salim et al, "Thymoquinone Induces Mitochondria-Mediated Apoptosis in Acute Lymphoblastic Leukemia in Vitro", Molecular Diversity Preservation International, https://www.mdpi.com/1420-3049/18/9/11219

[109] Rajput S et al, "Molecular targeting of Akt by thymoquinone promotes G(1) arrest through translation inhibition of cyclin D1 and induces apoptosis in breast cancer cells", US National Library of Medicine, https://www.ncbi.nlm.nih.gov/pubmed/24044882

[110] Hamed MA et al, "Effects of black seed oil on resolution of hepato-renal toxicity induced by bromobenzene in rats", US National Library of Medicine, https://www.ncbi.nlm.nih.gov/pubmed/23543440

[111] Murli L. Mathur et al, "Antidiabetic Properties of a Spice Plant Nigella Sativa", Journal of Endocrinology & Metabolism, https://www.jofem.org/index.php/jofem/article/viewArticle/15/15

Finally, a placebo-controlled clinical trial found that black seed oil can increase sperm count and improve sperm movement.[112]

Vegetables and Herbs

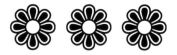

وكان صلى الله عليه وآله وسلم يأكل القثاء بالملح ، ويأكل البطيخ بالجبن ، ويأكل الفاكهة الرطبة ، وربما أكل البطيخ باليدين جميعاً .

He ﷺ would eat cucumber with salt and eat melon with cheese. He would eat fresh fruit, and would sometimes eat watermelon with both hands.

Some leading food writers have noted that salting cucumbers is a good way to retain its juices.[113] [114]

The combination of opposite foods is a common feature in traditional medicines – this may be why the Prophet linked certain foods.

وقال صلى الله عليه وآله وسلم : كلوا الثوم فان فيها شفاء من سبعين داء.

The Prophet ﷺ said, "Eat garlic, for in it is the remedy for seventy maladies."

It is recommended to abstain from the mosque after eating garlic due to its smell. The Prophet said, "He who eats this plant should not go to our mosque, nor should he harm us with the odour of garlic." (مَنْ أَكَلَ مِنْ هَذِهِ

الشَّجَرَةِ فَلاَ يَقْرَبَنَّ مَسْجِدَنَا وَلاَ يُؤْذِيَنَّا بِرِيحِ الثُّومِ)

[113] Mark Bittman, "The Minimalist; How Salting Cucumbers Works Magic in a Dish", The New York Times,
https://www.nytimes.com/1998/07/08/dining/the-minimalist-how-salting-cucumbers-works-magic-in-a-dish.html
[114] L.V Anderson, "You're Doing It Wrong: Cucumbers", Slate,
https://slate.com/culture/2013/08/salting-cucumbers-why-you-should-always-do-it-especially-for-tzatziki.html

Garlic is used for a wide range of conditions linked to the bloodstream and heart, including atherosclerosis, high cholesterol, heart disease, and hypertension.[115]

According to a controlled study conducted at the Jiangsu Provincial Center for Disease Control and Prevention, those who ate raw garlic twice a week over a seven-year period were 44% less likely to develop lung cancer.[116]

One study suggests that organo-sulfur compounds found in garlic have been identified as effective in destroying the cells in glioblastomas, a deadly type of brain tumour.[117]

Women whose diets are rich in allium vegetables, which include garlic, leeks, shallots, and onions, are reported to have lower levels of osteoarthritis.[118]

Diallyl sulfide, a compound in garlic, was 100 times more effective than two popular antibiotics in fighting the

[115] Tim Newman, "What are the benefits of garlic?", Medical News Today, https://www.medicalnewstoday.com/articles/265853#uses
[116] Zi-Yi Jin et al, "Raw Garlic Consumption as a Protective Factor for Lung Cancer, a Population-Based Case-Control Study in a Chinese Population", American Association for Cancer Research, https://cancerpreventionresearch.aacrjournals.org/content/6/7/711?sid=179e57a9-3770-409d-84bc-cd83ef816963
[117] Arabinda Das et al, "Garlic compounds generate reactive oxygen species leading to activation of stress kinases and cysteine proteases for apoptosis in human glioblastoma T98G and U87MG cells", American Cancer Society, https://acsjournals.onlinelibrary.wiley.com/doi/full/10.1002/cncr.22888
[118] Frances MK Williams et al, "Dietary garlic and hip osteoarthritis: evidence of a protective effect and putative mechanism of action", BioMed Central, https://bmcmusculoskeletdisord.biomedcentral.com/articles/10.1186/1471-2474-11-280

Campylobacter bacterium, according to a study published in the Journal of Antimicrobial Chemotherapy.[119]

Researchers at Ankara University investigated the effects of garlic extract supplementation on the blood lipid (fat) profile of patients with high blood cholesterol. Their study was published in the Journal of Nutritional Biochemistry.[120]

A 2013 study published in the Asian Pacific Journal of Cancer Prevention concluded that allium vegetables, especially garlic, are related to a decreased risk of prostate cancer.[121]

وقال صلى الله عليه وآله وسلم : من اكل السداب ونام عليه أمن من الدوار وذات الجنب .

---

[119] "Garlic compound fights source of food-borne illness", Washington state University, https://news.wsu.edu/2012/05/01/garlic-compound-fights-source-of-food-borne-illness/

[120] Ilker Durak et al, "Effects of garlic extract consumption on blood lipid and oxidant/antioxidant parameters in humans with high blood cholesterol", Science Direct, https://www.sciencedirect.com/science/article/abs/pii/S095528630400403

[121] Xiao-Feng Zhou et al, "Allium Vegetables and Risk of Prostate Cancer: Evidence from 132,192 Subjects", Korea Science, http://www.koreascience.or.kr/article/JAKO201332479511825.page

The Prophet ﷺ said, "One who eats rue, and sleeps upon it, is secure from vertigo (*ad-duwār*) and pleurisy (*dhāt al-janb*)."

Rue has been used in the treatment of disorders of the nervous system such as multiple sclerosis and Bell's palsy, as well as in curing dizziness and vertigo.[122]

Rue is also used for breathing problems including pain and coughing due to swelling around the lungs (pleurisy).[123]

وقال صلى الله عليه وآله وسلم : إذا دخلتم بلداً فكلوا من بقله او بصله يطرد عنكم داؤه ويذهب بالنصب ويشد العصب ويزيد في الباه ـ ويذهب بالحمى .

The Prophet ﷺ said, "When you enter a country, then eat of its vegetables or onions. It shall keep you from its malady, remove hardship, strengthen the nerve, increase in sexual potency, and get rid of fever."

---

[122] P.N. Ravindran et al, "Ruta graveolens", Science Direct, https://www.sciencedirect.com/topics/agricultural-and-biological-sciences/ruta-graveolens
[123] "Rue", WebMD, https://www.webmd.com/vitamins/ai/ingredientmono-885/rue

Every land has its own unique microbial ecosystem, and in a time before vaccines, one could become very ill simply by mixing into a new population. Hence, it is important to keep healthy whilst travelling. According to health expert Luke Coutinho, onions are the most powerful natural antibiotic; and they are a great treatment for colds, coughs, high fevers, and sore throats.[124] It include immune-boosting nutrients including vitamin C, zinc, selenium, and quercetin.

Onions' vitamin C content aids in healthy nerve function. It activates enzymes needed to make norepinephrine, a compound nerve cells need to communicate. Adding onions to one's diet also increases one's intake of vitamin B6, or pyridoxine. Vitamin B6 is used to metabolize glucose, the primary source of fuel for nerve cells. Onions introduce more manganese into one's diet, which benefits the nerves. Manganese benefits brain health by converting a potentially toxic compound called glutamate into a less toxic substance called GABA.[125]

Onion is considered a natural aphrodisiac as it increases testosterone in men, thereby increasing their libido.[126]

[124] "You Can Get Rid of Common Cold and Cough By Drinking Onion Juice! Health Expert Luke Coutinho Tells Us All About It", NDTV, https://www.ndtv.com/health/get-rid-of-common-cold-and-cough-by-drinking-onion-juice-health-expert-luke-coutinho-suggests-other-1939103

[125] Sylvie Tremblay, "Are Onions Good for the Nerves?" SFGate, https://healthyeating.sfgate.com/onions-good-nerves-10595.html

[126] Saleem Ali Banihani, "Testosterone in Males as Enhanced by Onion", US National Library of Medicine, https://www.ncbi.nlm.nih.gov/pmc/articles/PMC6406961/

وقال صلى الله عليه وآله وسلم : عليكم بالكرفس فانه ان كان شيء

يزيد في العقل فهو هو .

The Prophet ﷺ said, "Eat celery, for if there is a
thing that increases the intellect, then it is it."

A 2010 study published in the Journal of Nutrition
reports that luteolin, a compound in celery, reduces age-
related inflammation in the brain and related memory
deficits by directly inhibiting the release of inflammatory
molecules in the brain.[127]

Celery can also reduce brain fog (mental fatigue),
because it contains sodium cluster salts that attach to
viral neurotoxins, disarming them.[128]

وقال صلى الله عليه وآله وسلم : لو كان في شيء شفاء لكان في

السناء.

---

[127] "Compound in celery, peppers reduces age-related memory
deficits", Science Daily,
https://www.sciencedaily.com/releases/2010/10/101013122601.htm
?fbclid=IwAR3ZcXe1TgzLgLsXu8emdrD5K64qowk7qgFOntAn0Q5lfp1V
BoWV7yWDUJM
[128] Anthony William, "How Celery Juice Helps Heal Brain Fog", Medical
Medium Blog, https://www.medicalmedium.com/blog/how-celery-
juice-helps-heal-brain-fog

The Prophet ﷺ said, "If there is healing in anything, then it is in senna."

There have been some case reports of people suffering from constipation, liver damage, coma or nerve damage after using senna. In these cases, people were using senna at much higher than the recommended doses and for more extended periods of time.[129]

Senna has anti-inflammatory and antiparasitic properties, and it is reportedly an effective laxative for constipation.[130] It is used for other conditions, including hemorrhoids and weight loss, [131] but there currently isn't enough research on the subject.

وقال صلى الله عليه وآله وسلم : عليكم بالاهليلج الاسود فانه من

شجر الجنة طعمه مر وفيه شفاء من كل داء .

The Prophet ﷺ said, "Upon you is the black myrobalan, for it is from the trees of Paradise. Its taste is bitter, and in it is treatment for every malady."

---

[129] Nicole Galan, "Is senna tea safe to drink?", Medical News Today, https://www.medicalnewstoday.com/articles/320659
[130] Ana Gotter, "What Is Senna Tea?", Healthline, https://www.healthline.com/health/senna-tea
[131] Ibid.

Black myrobalan, also known as terminalia chebula, is a plant that has antibacterial qualities.[132] It contains biochemicals such as hydrolysable tannins, phenolic compounds, and flavonoids. Its antioxidant and anti-inflammatory effects make it an effective way to treat Alzheimer's.[133]

It possesses multiple pharmacological and medicinal activities, making it antidiabetic, hepatoprotective, radioprotective, cardioprotective, antirachitic, and even good for wound-healing.[134] Thus, it can be used in the treatment of diabetes, drug-induced liver damage, cardiovascular health, arthritis, and skincare.

Traditionally, black myrobalan has been used in Asia to treat asthma, sore throat, vomiting, ulcers, and many other conditions.[135]

Disclaimer: this is not a replacement for cancer or Alzheimer's treatment. Please speak to a physician and seek his or her recommendations in these matters.

---

[132] Malekzadeh F, "Antibacterial activity of black myrobalan (Terminalia chebula Retz) against Helicobacter pylori", US National Library of Health, https://www.ncbi.nlm.nih.gov/pubmed/11463533
[133] Amir R. Afshari et al, "A Review on Potential Mechanisms of Terminalia chebula in Alzheimer's Disease", US National Library of Medicine, https://www.ncbi.nlm.nih.gov/pmc/articles/PMC4749770/
[134] Anwesa Bag et al, "The development of Terminalia chebula Retz. (Combretaceae) in clinical research", US National Library of Medicine, https://www.ncbi.nlm.nih.gov/pmc/articles/PMC3631759/
[135] Ibid.

CONCLUSIONS

As I have demonstrated, there is much contemporary benefit that can be found in traditional Islamic medicinal texts. Of course, one must not neglect any aspect of the Sunna, whether or not it is supported by modern studies. Presuppositionless logic and intuition brings one to God; thereafter, one must entrust oneself to God and His commandments.

Future research on this topic could:

- Analyze other books in this genre.
- Offer a proper *taḥqīq* of the narrations included in this book.
- Produce controlled studies or meta-analyses on the foods mentioned in this book and their intended uses.
- Produce meal plans that incorporates foods prescribed in this genre of literature.
- Elaborate on the ethical and symbolic dimensions of the foods mentioned in this genre.
- Compare and contrast prophetic medicine to other forms of traditional medicine.

Allah is the Infinite, who heals our ills through the finite.

وآخر دعوانا أن الحمد لله رب العالمين

Printed in Great Britain
by Amazon